To Diane,
May all your plans
be good ones!
I am so proud of you.
Can't wait to call
you Dr. Diane!
♡
Mari

PRAISE FOR *Mair Hill*

As I have said before and undoubtedly will say again, you have single handedly changed my life and have made me believe in myself and cheered me onto business victory (still can't believe I won!) You have also cheered me on in personal matters and have guided me and led me and instructed me. I am eternally blessed and humbled and oh so grateful for your presence in my life.

-Helen K. Feykes

I am beyond grateful that my path crossed with Mair's. Mair's joyful, intuitive and direct approach made it easy for me to look into the mirror, so to speak, and see all of the possibilities reflected back at me. From the basics to the more complex, Mair guided me toward a happier, more fulfilling path. We started with my language and shifted it from the negative to the positive. We examined what I wanted and who I wanted to be, and Mair taught me to focus on the 'why' and to trust that I had the tools to handle the 'how'. I was at a crossroad with my career when I met Mair, and I am thrilled to say that my career and my business are flourishing. Everyone needs a Mair in their life – she is a game changer.

-Karen Collins

The health choice levels are well laid out. Each person can find a choice level that fits their capability. Many plans tell you if want to get healthy you must follow the one plan specified in the book, which for many, is unrealistic.

-Dino Sirakides

A Good Plan is a simple, fresh, and easy approach to becoming the healthiest version of yourself! Mair breaks it down to "good, better and best" offering something for everyone. I like that the reader can feel supported wherever they are starting. The Good Plan clearly defines clear cut steps to continue to dive further into one's wellness journey. Mair provides good resources and insight to get you on your way. As an allied health professional with over 25 years in the industry, I will definitely recommend this book to my patients.

-Kelly Kurtz

With this update, Mair Hill has brought together new facts and fresh ideas while ensuring her book is still a practical, easy-to-follow guide for a healthier lifestyle. I found her format of Good-Better-Best useful to implement because I never felt overwhelmed while following her advice. I am certain you will too.

-Jeanette McCauley

Mair Hill states that you know it all. You know what to do to get healthier... eat more veggies, less red meat, exercise a little more, BUT she also says that sometimes it is like we speak a different language and we don't quite understand. With the motto 'One Size Doesn't Fit All,' Mair approaches the goals of her readers to find a balance to their health and well-being. She offers a 10-step plan: beginning with the right mindset, the basic eating, sleep, water, etc. she really visits subjects we all know. However, she adds her own twist, which makes it easy understandable and workable for all of us. "A Good Plan" really is what the title promises.

-Alexandra Roach

A Good Plan is just that, a clever way to approach getting good, better or the best health plan. Mair gives you options depending on just how much you want to put forward. I like that she has included some charts with helpful information to make my plan work the best for me! I am looking forward to working my plan!

-Martie Pineda

Wow! Fast. Breezy. Concise. Mair's writing style is wildly efficient. She packs so much information on each page that if you blink you might miss something! This is a book you can get through fast and yet you'll want to reread it just to make sure you absorb everything. It's also a book you'll want to keep around as a reminder of how and what to do. I guess that's the point - It's a good plan and a great job Mair.

-Rich Hill

A GOOD PLAN

A
GOOD PLAN

INTENTIONALLY SIMPLE

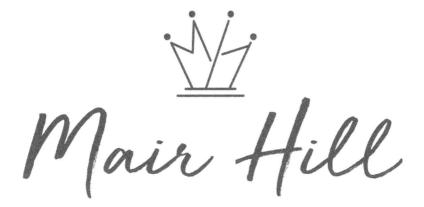

BALBOA.
PRESS

A DIVISION OF HAY HOUSE

Balboa Press books may be ordered through booksellers or by contacting:

Balboa Press
A Division of Hay House
1663 Liberty Drive
Bloomington, IN 47403
www.balboapress.com
1 (877) 407-4847

Because of the dynamic nature of the Internet, any web addresses or links contained in this book may have changed since publication and may no longer be valid. The views expressed in this work are solely those of the author and do not necessarily reflect the views of the publisher, and the publisher hereby disclaims any responsibility for them.

The author of this book does not dispense medical advice or prescribe the use of any technique as a form of treatment for physical, emotional, or medical problems without the advice of a physician, either directly or indirectly. The intent of the author is only to offer information of a general nature to help you in your quest for emotional and spiritual well-being. In the event you use any of the information in this book for yourself, which is your constitutional right, the author and the publisher assume no responsibility for your actions.

Any people depicted in stock imagery provided by Getty Images are models, and such images are being used for illustrative purposes only. Certain stock imagery © Getty Images.

Photo by Lynn Renee Photography

Print information available on the last page.

ISBN: 978-1-9822-3640-3 (sc)
ISBN: 978-1-9822-3642-7 (hc)
ISBN: 978-1-9822-3641-0 (e)

Library of Congress Control Number: 2019915761

Balboa Press rev. date: 10/11/2019

For my Mom and Dad
who always taught me
I could do anything

And for Rich
who supported me as I did

Wellness is the Conscious,
Deliberate and Self-Directed
Pursuit of Living Life
to its
Fullest Potential

Mair Hill

YOU. ONLY BETTER.
Personally. Professionally. Energetically.

CONTENTS

Are you tired of being tired and sick of being sick?

Do you believe being healthy requires more time and effort than you have – or are willing to give? Are you overwhelmed with all the conflicting advice that's currently available?

Welcome to A GOOD PLAN!

A GOOD PLAN is a primer. It's designed to get you started. To inspire you to make incremental changes at your own pace. Simple. Easy. Doable. That's the best way to incorporate them into your daily life. To create a healthy lifestyle.

There is no one-size-fits-all program. That's why each Step in A GOOD PLAN is broken down into GOOD, BETTER, BEST recommendations so no matter where you are today, you have the perfect place to start.

When you follow these Best practices, you will have an overall sense of wellness, more energy, better productivity and sustained happiness. You may even drop a few pounds far easier than you have in the past.

All you have to do is open the book and begin.

PREFACE

A few years ago, my husband and I traveled to Australia for the first time to attend the wedding of a friend of mine. We started our trip in Sydney. On the second day we took the train to one of the seaside towns, called Bondi, to have lunch. My friend had recommended a nice seafood restaurant. It was late in the afternoon and we were the only ones in this restaurant on a dreary, random, Thursday in September, which is the beginning of their spring.

We were still jet-lagged and not yet accustomed to the Australian accent. Our very tall waiter handed each of us a menu and then proceeded to tell us about the fish specials for the day. When he was done, I just looked at him and said, "I'm sorry, I didn't understand a word you just said."

He paused, leaned over, got really close to my face, and speaking slowly and loudly, said,

"WHAT KIND OF FISH DO YOU WANT?"

I tell you that story because perhaps that's how you will "hear" some of what I will present to you in this book – like I'm speaking a foreign language. Even though it's in English, much like the Australian waiter's speech, the "accent" may be different than what you're used to hearing.

My goal is to present new ways of thinking about stuff that you already know. Of course, you do! Everyone knows they need to eat more vegetables and fruits, eat less red meat, eat less sugar and exercise more. But what exactly does that mean? What exactly does that look like? How much, exactly, is more? And most importantly, how do you fit all of that into your very busy, already-too-full, everyday life?

I applaud you and honor you for picking up this book. You must be ready for a change (or at the very least, seriously thinking about it!). You must be ready to feel better in all areas of your life. YAY! You've come to the right place. My mission is to empower YOU to take care of YOU. A vibrant life, lived in a healthy lifestyle, is waiting.

What follows are ten simple Steps that are so easy you will actually do them. Right? Because knowing and doing are two very different things. Unless, and until, you start incorporating some healthier habits, not only will your health **not** improve, it may even get worse.

I believe to improve your overall health and wellness, what you eat is more important than exercising. Of course exercise is one of the ten Steps because moving your body is vital to keeping all your parts working smoothly, but I hope it's a relief for those of you who don't like to exercise to know that you are not expected to run a marathon in order to achieve better health.

It will be up to you to decide what's right for you and what will fit into your life now, maybe next week, maybe next year, maybe never. A GOOD PLAN is one you can do and as you try on these new techniques, some will fit naturally and just become part of your daily wardrobe. Like brushing your teeth. You won't even have to think about them anymore because they will just become habit. Some may require a little tailoring before they fit perfectly. These ten simple Steps are recommendations. Suggestions for ways to just begin. Easily. I'm all about simple!

Because we're all different, there is no one-size-fits-all plan. With each of these ten Steps, I provide a GOOD, BETTER, and BEST option since we're not all starting from the same place. At the end of each Step, I even include an INTENTIONALLY SIMPLE suggestion to really get your motivation flowing. Each of these Steps will have a different priority in your current lifestyle.

No doubt, in some areas you will already be at the BEST level. Yay for you! That means you can focus on starting at GOOD on a different Step. Over time, as you move closer to the BEST in every Step, your health will improve so dramatically, you will forget where you started. Your new, healthy lifestyle will allow you to live a vibrant life.

I get asked all the time how I know this stuff. I have been living a wellness lifestyle for decades. I live and breathe these ten Steps so naturally, sometimes I forget not everyone lives this way. I want to change that!

I graduated from Colby College and after running my own sales agency for seventeen years, I went back to school to study nutrition. I am now a Certified Holistic Health Coach, Reiki Master and Professional Speaker. I run workshops in wellness and personal transformation along with a small private practice where I get to work with clients one-on-one.

And now I am here with you to share Intentionally Simple ways to create your own GOOD PLAN. My promise to you: when you follow these Best practices, you will experience a better overall sense of wellness, increased energy, more productivity and sustained happiness. You may even drop a few pounds far easier than you ever thought possible.

I am not a doctor. I won't get all science-y on you. This book is a primer: a simple, easy, and effective way to get started on a healthier path. If you want deeper knowledge and understanding on any of these subjects, I encourage you to explore them further on your own.

There are also additional recommendations and resources available on my website: www.mairhill.com.

One of my favorite Zen expressions is:
when the student is ready, the teacher will appear.

I know you are ready.
I am truly honored to be your teacher.

Mair Hill
Chicago, 2019

INTRODUCTION

This book is all about you. All for you. Even if you are caring for young children or aging parents or a significant other, YOU are still the best person to take care of YOU. There's a reason the airlines tell you to put your oxygen mask on first. You can't take care of anyone else, unless you are healthy yourself. Without a healthy you, those that depend on you will suffer too.

Let's start with what YOU believe. All those thoughts running around in your head. Whether you're aware of them or not, they all matter. Every single one of them. All the time. Not only your thoughts, but your awareness of them. When we go through life on autopilot, not only do we miss the joys along the way – both big and small - but we may end up somewhere we don't want to be. To maximize the effectiveness of this ten Step plan, we must start with your head.

I could tell you to eat kale at every meal, but unless you are ready for, and committed to, change, all the kale in the world won't matter. The fact that you're reading this book is an excellent start, but it needs to go further. You need to make **YOU** a priority and commit to actually taking the Steps outlined here.

My husband, Rich, is the perfect example. With his permission, I'm going to share his story. He could always eat anything he wanted and not gain a pound. Until he turned thirty. After that, his bloodwork numbers* were less than stellar. Since he has some genetic stuff that runs in his family (and because he is, by training, an engineer), he has kept a spreadsheet for the past twenty years that lists all his biometric numbers. This amazing spreadsheet includes a column noting any significant aberrations.

He's tried to blame his poor test results on genetics and yet he knows that when he eats properly, his numbers improve enough to put him in the normal range. When he has agreed to do a diet detox with me or when he gave up drinking beer, the results were fairly quick and very dramatic: normal. But when he went back to his old ways, his numbers returned to the unhealthy range. It was very clear that diet mattered.

Rich would always tell me I am in the 99th percentile. He would say most people were just not willing to do what I do or were as disciplined, etc. So instead, he would watch me eat healthy foods, avoid coffee and alcohol, skip dessert and then he would continue to eat what he wanted. Finally, his doctor started making noise about taking a statin drug to get his numbers into a healthier range. Rich was not ready to start taking prescription drugs.

The only compromise Rich was willing to make was to see a registered dietician. Yes, it's true, he paid money for a third party to tell him how to eat. When he got home from his first (and only) appointment, I asked what the dietician said, and he admitted it was everything I had already told him. In the end, he didn't take her advice any more than he took mine.

Soon after that, Rich finally agreed to follow his doctor's advice and started taking a statin drug. He didn't get the benefits he wanted, and he didn't love the way it made him feel physically so he was (finally) ready to try it my way. He was ready to commit to making himself a

---

* By "numbers" I am referring to some standard markers the medical community uses to assess your health: cholesterol (both HDL & LDL), triglycerides, glucose and blood pressure. To protect Rich's privacy, I am not revealing which numbers were affected.

priority. He was ready to put his oxygen mask on first. He was ready to change.

I have more than one hundred diet and eating-right type books. I prefer to follow a plan – if someone else was willing to figure it out for me, all the better! I would dive into these books and I would last a while but for the most part, these plans are not what I call real life. If a GOOD PLAN is something you can do, then it's important to find what fits your lifestyle.

Rich found that plan. For him it was based on one of those books. But in the end, he made it his own and he stuck to it. He lost over twenty pounds and more importantly, his numbers improved to again put him in the normal range, without any medication.

I can help you do this too.

HOW TO USE THIS BOOK

Use this book as a primer. It's designed to be an introduction to a healthier way of life. Ideally you would start at the beginning and read all the way through to the end. But, if you're like me, the temptation will be to skip to the exact Step that interests you most. That's okay if you agree to read the first Step on Mindset. To make the most of the rest of the Steps and take full advantage of the very simple wisdom in this book, you need to start at the beginning: Step 1 – Mindset.

The GOOD, BETTER and BEST options all build on the one preceding it. So, if you start at GOOD and realize it's already part of your daily routine, skip ahead to BETTER. However, please only continue to BETTER once you've at least attempted GOOD. For the simplest way to begin one of the Steps – skip to the end of the chapter and start with INTENTIONALLY SIMPLE.

This book is designed to inspire you to make incremental changes at your own pace. Simple. Easy. Doable. That's the best way to incorporate them into your daily life. That's the best way to make permanent changes until a healthy lifestyle is a habit.

My hope is once you master all the BEST practices here and understand what it's like to feel really good every single day that you will never want to go back to where you began.

Slow and steady wins the race.

This "race" is your vibrant, energetic, healthy life.

STEP 1

Mindset

Whether you think you can or think you can't, you will be right.
-Henry Ford

What you think matters. You get more of what you think about: both positive and negative. When you commit to a change, or a project, or a new direction, in the words of Paulo Coelho in *The Alchemist,* "the whole universe conspires to help you." It all begins in your mind with the words you use, not only when you're speaking to someone, but even more importantly, when you are talking to yourself.

When you set a deliberate intention, you will be amazed at the people that show up in your life at the "perfect" time; at the articles that will "suddenly" appear in your in box; at the things you will see for the "first" time that were in front of you all along. All you have to do is articulate your desire and then "the whole universe" will indeed set in motion everything you need.

My husband, again, is the perfect example. He wanted his biometric numbers to be better, but in the beginning, he was not willing to commit to improving his diet. Remember, what you eat is more important than exercise when it comes to improving your health markers.

Once he decided, really decided, he was ready, everything fell into place. He was ready to let me help him. He stopped playing the "poor me-I'm-not-allowed-to-eat-anything-good-any-more" card and started to eat food that nourished him properly. He stopped craving junk food before going to sleep, which meant that he woke up easier and had better energy during the day. The benefits kept mounting. Before he knew it, he lost twenty pounds and all of his biometric numbers were in the normal range. With very little effort.

I promise I can do the same for you, but first, you need to make the commitment. To you. Not me. YOU are making the commitment to YOU!

I believe anyone can run a marathon. My husband will argue that not everyone *wants* to run a marathon. That's a different discussion. Running a marathon is a mental game, just like getting healthy. I was never a runner. When someone challenged me to run my first 5k, I argued for a while (truly, I never even liked running!) but I thought about it. Then I thought some more. Finally, I decided to accept the challenge.

I didn't even know how far 5k was (3.1 miles). In my own methodical way, I went about training for my first 5k. I measured the distance. I bought the right shoes. I read a book on running. After that first race, I was hooked! I loved the feeling of accomplishment. I loved the energy of all the people participating in the race.

A few months later, a friend suggested I train for a half marathon. I didn't know such a thing existed and once again, I had no idea how far a half marathon was (13.1 miles). Once I accomplished that, I set my sights on the Chicago Marathon the following year. I joined a running group and committed to the training.

Training meant more than just logging the miles every week. It included a huge mental component. It meant committing the time to run several times per week. That required rearranging my schedule accordingly. It meant eating properly to fuel my body for those long runs. Drinking plenty of water to hydrate. Going to bed on time to be sure my body had enough time to rest and repair. Which meant making the training a priority over my social life.

And it all started with my desire. Wanting to. Believing I could. Knowing I could.

Creating a healthy lifestyle requires the same commitment: thinking about it, being willing to rearrange your priorities and taking the time to do what's necessary. Once you do, you'll be hooked! You won't believe how good you will feel. You'll be amazed at your new-found energy.

In the following pages, I have laid out your own personal plan. A GOOD PLAN. Maybe you aren't running an actual marathon, but when you have achieved the best practices of these ten Steps, you will feel equally as accomplished as I did when I finished those 26.2 miles.

Ready? Let's start at the beginning.

Mindset - Good

The beginning is awareness. Awareness of your surroundings. Awareness of what you're thinking. Awareness of what you're eating. Take notice of what you're doing. Get into the habit of just checking in with yourself. Get to know your body. You're in it. No one else can know better than you how your body feels when you are stressed, when you eat, when you have slept well (or not!), when you walk, when you laugh, etc.

Your awareness will serve you well once you start making changes. You'll better understand that when you do THIS, then THAT happens. Cause and effect. You'll then be able to make educated choices.

Be present. Right here. Right now. That's especially important when you're eating. It's really easy to eat mindlessly and before you know it, you've inhaled your dinner without even tasting a bite. (Or worse a bag of potato chips or a pint of ice cream while watching television. How sad to miss out on all the pleasure from consuming all those calories. Without being present, you do not even taste what you're eating!)

Have you ever been driving and once you arrived at your destination, you realized you don't remember anything about your route? That's truly being on autopilot. That can be terrifying – and dangerous – especially when you're behind the wheel of a car.

Autopilot can also lead to sadness and regret when you've been doing something you normally enjoy, but don't reap the benefits because your mind is somewhere else. (Think back to that bag of potato chips or pint of ice cream...)

Practice being present. Skip thinking about the items left undone on your TO-DO list or worrying about whether you did the wrong thing this morning. Just be right here. Right now.

Mindset – Better

Once you're aware of what you're thinking, saying, and eating, you can start affecting the changes you want. As you start to become aware, when you check in with yourself, start asking yourself 'what do I want?' Practice noticing how you feel about what you're doing. What you're eating. Are you enjoying it? If not, ask yourself what would make it better? Allow yourself the time to answer that question – what would make it better? What would you rather be doing? If you're already enjoying it, acknowledge that too. Say thank you. Out loud. Often.

Start thinking/saying/eating what you do want, instead of what you don't want. Here's a simple example, let's say you have a big outdoor activity planned for this weekend. Instead of thinking 'I don't want it to rain' because that is exactly what you DON'T want; think instead what you DO want: clear skies and sunshine. Do you want to remember to take your keys with you when you leave the house? Or would you rather not forget them? This is very subtle, but very powerful. And very simple. Every time you hear yourself saying the word DON'T, pause and reword your statement to reflect what you DO want.

Sometimes that will require a bit of thinking since the opposite is not always true. For example, if you don't want to go down, it doesn't mean you necessarily want to go up, it might simply mean you want to go over there. Make sense?

First you need to be aware of what you're thinking and then you can commit to practicing changing your focus.

Now that you're aware of what you're thinking, you'll notice that when you focus on what you do want, it feels much better than focusing on something you don't. It's like telling someone to not think about pink elephants. Chances are, for at least the next several minutes, you'll be thinking about pink elephants.

Here's a better real-life example - you've just committed to getting healthier and someone presents you with a piece chocolate cake. Or a pint of your favorite ice cream, or chips and guacamole or [insert your favorite junk food here], what do you do?

If you say I don't want the chocolate cake. I don't want the chocolate cake. I don't want the chocolate cake. Not only will you keep thinking about the chocolate cake, you will probably eat a lot more of it, or worse yet, binge on something else if the chocolate cake is no longer available. It would have been a lot easier – and more beneficial, had you just asked yourself the following question:

'Do I really want to eat this chocolate cake?'

Then, using everything you're practicing in this BETTER section of Mindset, if the answer is yes, then do it! Be present so you will taste every bite. Give yourself permission to eat it and enjoy it! Guilt free.

We'll talk a little later about the best way to eat the chocolate cake.

Mindset - Best

At this level you're aware and you have started to focus on what you do want instead of what you don't. You're aware of the way you feel when you're thinking/saying/eating something you do want. Your brain does not know if what you're telling it is the truth or a lie, and it will accommodate you accordingly. If you continue to lament that you're overweight or you have high blood pressure, the daily circumstances that present themselves to you will make sure you're right. You are indeed overweight. You do indeed have high blood pressure.

Practice being right about what you want to be right about.

Worth noting, it just feels better to think kind thoughts – about yourself and others. You wouldn't tell your best friend that she's fat, so why would you say that to yourself?

Repeat after me: I'm great! I'm awesome! I'm loving and loveable! Keep repeating it until these words feel natural to you and it literally puts a smile on your face and creates lightness in your heart.

With all your new awareness, you've changed the way you think. The way you talk. Now the fun begins! As you do these things, you will be inspired to do more. It's called deliberate action. It's the way "the whole universe conspires to help you" once you set an intention. When you set that intention, you will be inspired to pick up the phone and call someone right now or turn right instead of left or read a certain article. Best of all, it will seem effortless!

Once you set your intention to create and live a healthy lifestyle and start focusing on what you DO want, all the rest of the pieces will naturally fall into place. Thinking about a healthy lunch will actually create the time you need to prepare it and take it with you to work (or someone may even just surprise you with a fresh garden salad!)

Saying you want to sleep better will make it easier to go to bed on time. Deliberately focusing on drinking more water will make water more available to you (it may seem that everywhere you go people will start offering you a glass of water).

Be aware of what transpires after you set your intention. The situations, people, articles and other resources that show up will astound you.

Mindset – Intentionally Simple

Take a moment right now to check in with the thoughts in your head. That on-going chatter that fills your mind. What are you saying? Are you being kind to yourself? Are you worried about something? Does what you're thinking feel good?

Being conscious is the first step to being deliberate. Once you are aware of what you're thinking, it's easier to change the chatter. Remember, you get to choose. If you don't like what you're hearing, choose words that feel better. Don't know what to say? How about a simple mantra like "I love myself" or "I'm so excited for what's coming" or "I'm grateful to be right here, right now."

When I'm feeling over-whelmed with a TO-DO list longer than there are minutes in the day, I love to say, "Time expands to meet my needs."

If your negative chatter dominates your thoughts, take back control with a few, feel-good words of your choosing. Write them down, keep them with you, until silently repeating them becomes your new habit.

NOTES

STEP 2

Eating Basics

Timing is everything.
-Unknown

In Step 1, I used chocolate cake to represent a food weakness, an indulgence; a food typically considered "bad." Yours could be ice cream or chips and guacamole, but for simplicity and consistency, I am just going to talk about chocolate cake. When do you get to eat your sugar indulgence? Remember we're creating a GOOD PLAN. A real-life plan. My real-life plan includes chocolate cake – what about yours?

I often read about (thin) celebrities saying they eat healthy all week and then have a "cheat" day. I've tried that before, but I found that if I arbitrarily designate Saturday as my "cheat" day, and the chocolate cake is offered to me on Wednesday – then what? If I eat the chocolate cake because it's available to me now, but might not be available again on Saturday, then is Wednesday my "cheat" day for the week? What if I ate healthy all-day Wednesday and the cake didn't appear until 6:00 p.m.? Did I "cheat" myself out of a "cheat" day because I could have been eating junk since the moment I got up on Wednesday morning, but didn't know it until 6:00 p.m. when the chocolate cake showed up?

Are you an over-thinker, like me?

Worse than just feeling overly complicated, it took the joy out of eating the chocolate cake. That's what we talked about in Step 1: if you're going to eat the cake, enjoy it!

In Step 1 we also talked about cultivating awareness of what you're thinking/saying/eating. Are you like most people – are you aware that you typically categorize chocolate cake as "bad" and that eating it constitutes "cheating"? With that awareness, you now have the power to choose a new way of thinking about chocolate cake. Without labels. To me, labels like "bad" and "cheat" suggest shame and frankly, they don't feel very good. Besides, we always want what we can't have, so saying you shouldn't eat the chocolate cake will only make you want it more. Remove the label.

Try thinking of chocolate cake like you think about toast or a turkey sandwich or anything else that is just neutral. And, like a turkey sandwich, chocolate cake can be included in your real-life plan. You just need to know the optimum time to eat it.

Eating Basics – Good

If you want to eat the chocolate cake, just to be sure to eat healthier stuff first and by healthier, I mean food that will nourish your body and your brain. (Any way you slice it, you will not derive the same nutritional benefits from eating chocolate cake as you would by eating a kale salad. To suggest otherwise would be misleading.)

When you eat a beautiful salad or an assortment of vegetables or lean protein first, you are simply feeding your body well before you eat the chocolate cake. You might even crowd out room in your stomach for that chocolate cake. Maybe, after eating a salad, a small slice of chocolate cake or even just a few bites will be enough to satisfy. If you want the chocolate cake, try eating an apple or drinking a glass of water, first.

Using the Mindset techniques from Step 1, while you're eating the apple or the salad, be aware of what you're eating. Be present. Right here. Right now.

Take a bite of whatever you're eating and chew it at least 15-20 times. Feel the texture in your mouth and really notice the taste and the flavor of what you're eating. Put down your fork between bites.

Chewing your food will give your digestive tract a head start – remember your stomach doesn't have teeth. The act of digesting your food takes more energy than anything else your body does, so chewing it well before you swallow it will free up all that extra energy.

Another advantage of taking time to really chew your food is that it takes twenty minutes for your brain to send the message to your belly that you're full. Twenty minutes! When is the last time it took you twenty minutes to eat your lunch? If you just inhale your food, especially if you are eating calorie-laden carbohydrates with a side of fat, you can literally eat the equivalent of several days' worth of calories by the time your belly sends a message to your brain to stop eating. You're full! If, after doing all this, you still want the chocolate cake, eat some. Chew it. Taste it. Enjoy it.

Eating Basics – Better

Remember each one of these sections builds on the last. So once being aware of what you're eating and chewing more thoroughly is a habit, then you can focus on a better way to eat that chocolate cake. You've asked yourself 'Do I want this chocolate cake?' and the answer is yes. You've eaten something healthier first and now you're ready to eat the chocolate cake.

BETTER is to cut off a slice of chocolate cake, put it on a plate and sit down at the table to eat it. Free of distractions. No television. No cell phone. Just you and your chocolate cake. Start with a small slice – you can always go back for more. If you want it.

Part of being aware is also being aware of what you want and not just mindlessly eating. Being aware of when your body is actually hungry (or full!) and honoring yourself enough to eat accordingly.

By putting a small slice of cake on a plate and sitting at the table to eat it, you will avoid standing at the fridge with the door open, fork in hand, grazing. Over-eating. Be present. It makes it easier to be aware of what you're eating.

Even BETTER would be to eat this sugar indulgence before 3:00 p.m. to allow your body to process it long before you go to sleep. I learned this in college – with iced tea (instead of chocolate cake, but truly both are stimulants to your system). If I drank the iced tea after 3:00 p.m., I had trouble falling asleep. Caffeine still affects me like that.

I have no scientific evidence regarding chocolate cake, but a friend of mine was getting sicker and sicker and no doctor could figure out what was wrong with her. She was already thin and getting thinner with no explanation. Finally, someone was insightful enough to inquire about her diet. Turns out she had a nightly ritual that started when she was a child: every night before she went to sleep, she ate milk and cookies. By the time she reached thirty, her body could no longer handle this ritual and she was waking up in what the doctors called a sugar coma. Once she stopped eating cookies before bed, all her symptoms disappeared.

I invite you to be aware of how you feel in the morning (especially after a good night's sleep). If you're still groggy, think about what you ate the night before and when you ate it. So many times, a restless night's sleep or sleeping well and still waking up groggy, is related to what you ate and when. The reverse is true too: when you eat a light, healthy dinner and nothing else before you go to sleep, you will sleep well and wake up refreshed.

I helped my youngest son with this. He is an athlete, so weight has never been a factor. e really liked eating a bowl of ice cream before bed. I never told him not to. Instead, when he started complaining about being tired in the morning, I asked him to think about what he ate the night before and when. He was able to see the correlation and as a result made his own informed decision to eat his ice cream earlier in the day.

It would be BETTER to eat the chocolate cake for breakfast (after a bowl of oatmeal or two scrambled eggs) than to eat it for desert after dinner.

Eating Basics - Best

The BEST practice continues with being aware of the timing of when you eat. We'll dive into what to eat in later Steps. First, I just want you to be aware of what you're eating and when you're eating it.

Ideally, you will eat within an hour of getting up to wake up your metabolism. Your metabolism helps regulate your body's systems by moving nutrients and hormones to where they are needed. It also helps your body burn calories. When you sleep, your metabolism naturally slows down to help your body do its best repair work. Exercising is another way to wake up your metabolism first thing in the morning (see Step 7).

Remember we are talking about BEST practices – not necessarily weight loss. The studies seem to be divided about eating breakfast and weight loss. Some say it's crucial to eat breakfast to keep you from bingeing at 3:00 p.m. with unhealthy carbs. Others say it really won't make a difference. Long term, however, is a different matter. The results are pretty consistent after several years: those who eat breakfast maintain their weight (and weight loss) easier than those who don't eat breakfast.

If you're not a breakfast eater – why is that? Not enough time? Too tired? These questions are worth answering for yourself. This book is about lifestyle changes – one simple Step at a time. You are where you are because of the choices you've made. To get somewhere new, you need to make new choices. One definition of insanity is to keep doing the same thing and expect different results. Without changing anything, next year you'll still be here, only probably worse.

Now that you've agreed to at least try to eat breakfast, the BEST practice is to stop eating at least three hours before going to bed. Nothing. I had a client ask me to be even more specific: she goes to bed at 10:30 p.m. but really doesn't fall asleep until midnight. She wanted to know if that meant she should stop eating at 7:30 p.m. or 9:00 p.m.? I have found it's easier to remember to just stop eating after 7:00 p.m.

So, what's the BEST eating practice between breakfast and 7:00 p.m.? Jorge Cruise wrote a book called *The Three-Hour Diet*. There's lots of science in it about insulin and hormones, but the basic premise is that when you eat every three hours, your body has a chance to fully digest and all systems will then be ready to handle more. Like a well-oiled machine. If you continually graze, you never let your body rest and recharge, so it has to work so much harder. It's like constantly revving your car engine. How long can it work that hard before it starts to breakdown?

Intermittent fasting follows this same idea – allowing your body plenty of time to rest. If you stop eating at 7:00 p.m. and wait until 7:00 a.m. before you eat again, you have effectively fasted for twelve hours.

Keeping all this in mind, an ideal day would be to wake up, eat within an hour and then eat every three hours after that, ending at 7:00 p.m. Remember that chocolate cake? If it's offered to you in the middle of those three hours, wait until the three-hour mark to eat it: after you've eaten the apple and before 3:00 p.m. You don't even have to really "remember" this – just set a reminder on your phone. Let it do the work for you.

If that seems complicated and overwhelming – please read it again. I have just given you a very simple way to eat. There's actually very little effort involved. It's all about your awareness – being aware of what you're eating and when. Sitting at your desk slowly devouring a bag of pretzels is completely mindless. You're on autopilot. You're probably not even deriving any pleasure from those pretzels. Nor are you honoring your body's signals about being hungry, or full.

Notice I have never said, don't eat the chocolate cake. To me that's not real life. And it has to be real life to be sustainable. I am just asking you to eat it mindfully - on purpose and with pleasure.

If this still just seems like a lot of rules, the label you give it is your choice and is totally subjective. How about calling it your new system? Or a recipe for great health? Only you can decide to improve. This book simply presents different levels within each Step: it's up to you to choose the ones you are willing to commit to incorporating into your lifestyle.

A GOOD PLAN is one you can do.

Eating Basics – Intentionally Simple

When was the last time you actually felt hungry? I had a client once who told me she ate because she thought she should. In other words, her mind told her to eat, instead of her body signaling it was time to eat. Allow yourself to get hungry. Get to know your body. It will tell you when you're hungry and equally as important, it will tell you when you're full.

NOTES

STEP 3

Sleep

A well-spent day brings happy sleep.
-Leonardo da Vinci

Sleep is delicious. Long before Arianna Huffington wrote *Thrive* and installed nap rooms in her corporate office, I encouraged the people who worked in my office to go into our conference room and take a 20-minute power nap. To be fully awake is to be fully functioning. More productive. More creative. Less stressed. Less likely to eat the donut for a pick-me-up. You already know that when you're sleepy, you're more easily irritated and less fun to be around.

According to the Mayo Clinic, when you are sleep deprived, you have an increased risk of high blood pressure. And high blood pressure has been linked to even more chronic diseases like stroke, dementia, kidney failure and a fatal heart attack. In short, chronic lack of sleep could equal death. Yikes!

Your body does its best repair work when you sleep. Your systems rest, renew, and balance out. It's like charging the battery on your cell phone. If you constantly unplug it before it's fully charged, you will shorten the lifespan of your battery. Fully charged means operating fully.

You have a greater risk of being obese when you don't get enough sleep. Research is on-going regarding the link between individuals who only sleep 5-6 hours per night and weight gain. It's not clear whether the pounds pile on because people are eating more doughnuts to compensate for lack of sleep or whether lack of sleep is somehow affecting their metabolism

Two key eating-related hormones rely on a good night's sleep: ghrelin which signals you're hungry and leptin which signals you're full. When these hormones get shut off or are not operating on full power, weight gain is sure to follow because no matter how much you eat, you never feel satisfied.

Lack of sleep will affect your job performance – whether your job is a student or salesperson or a full-time mom. One study found that college students who pull all-nighters to prepare for tests tend to have lower grade point averages than those who get regular sleep. Anytime you get behind the wheel of a car when you're sleepy, you run the risk of injuring not only yourself, but innocent people in your path.

Sleep needs to be a priority.

Sleep - Good

Melatonin helps regulate the sleep-wake cycle. It is a hormone your body makes naturally. Sometimes it can get disrupted or interrupted – like when you take a red-eye flight. That's why supplements are available to help you get back on track. However, on a day-to-day basis, your body naturally produces what you need. Especially when you help it. Bright light before bed has been shown to disrupt the production of melatonin. A GOOD practice is to power down at least one hour before bed. That includes television and electronic devices such as a computer, a tablet or a cell phone. This also helps you rest your mind and prepare it for sleep.

If the lighting in your bedroom is bright, install a dimmer on the switch for the overhead light. They are inexpensive and easy to install. Buy three-way bulbs for any lamps in your bedroom. If you keep a clock by your bed, buy one with the ability to dim the light on the face. If you need to have ambient light, try using a small night light, otherwise sleep in a dark room.

Charge your cell phone in another room.

Sleep - Better

Keep the same sleep hours. Your body loves routine. If you are diligent about going to bed at the same time every night, your body will know what to do. If you work a traditional full-time job, you are already an expert on half the equation: chances are, at least Monday through Friday, you get up at the same time every morning. To achieve this BETTER practice means also going to bed at the same time every night and keeping roughly the same hours on the weekend.

Without adequate sleep, you develop a sleep debt. A sleep debt is the amount of sleep you're getting versus the amount of sleep you need. You cannot make up for all the sleep you lost during the week by sleeping later on weekends.

Experts agree that most people need an average of 7-8 hours of sleep per night. A study by the National Sleep Foundation showed that on average, Americans get 6.8 hours of sleep per night during the week and 7.4 hours of sleep per night on weekends. That nightly sleep loss creates an annual sleep debt that adds up to more than two full weeks.

Sleep - Best

You can actually determine the ideal amount of sleep that's optimal for you. The 7-8 hours of sleep that most experts agree is the right amount, is just that – an average. That means the range is really somewhere between 6 and 9 hours of sleep per night – that's a big range! To determine where you fall in this range, you need to go to bed when you are sleepy and wake up naturally – without an alarm clock. Be aware of how you feel and honor your body when you are tired. You have about a 20-minute window to crawl into bed and fall asleep. After that you get your "second wind" and it may take a lot longer to fall asleep.

You may need to plan your personal sleep study for a vacation or a long weekend. In the beginning, you will probably be working off the accumulated sleep debt, but eventually you will discover the amount of sleep that is optimal for you. Until then, try going to bed a few minutes earlier each night until you are able to wake up feeling rested. Turning off all electronics at least one hour before bed and being aware of what you eat and when you eat it will make this process easier and more accurate.

So far, these first three Steps have really been about lifestyle changes. These are as important as what you eat for improving your overall health. Except for using chocolate cake as an example, I haven't even mentioned food. When you start mastering some of these Steps, and they just become part of your routine, the whole what-food-am-I-supposed-to-eat will get easier too.

Promise.

Sleep – Intentionally Simple

Use your bed for what it was designed for: sleep (and intimacy), instead of as an office or a snack table. Let your bed be your sanctuary. No computer, no phone, no potato chips or crackers or ice cream. When you train your body that crawling into bed means going to sleep, your body will learn that when you crawl into bed, you're there to sleep. And it will happen easier and faster.

NOTES

STEP 4

Water

Water is the driving force of all nature.
-Leonardo da Vinci

Before we dive into what to feed your body, we need to talk about something even more important: water. Water makes up 60% of our total body weight. We cannot survive more than a few days, maybe a week, without water, whereas, we can make it without food for several weeks. Mahatma Gandhi survived his 21-day hunger strike without food, but he did sip water.

Most of our important body parts and major organs are made of water: the brain and heart are 73% water; the lungs 83%; and even our bones are over 30% water. Skin, our largest and fastest growing organ, contains 64% water. Every muscle, joint, and cell in our bodies relies on water for optimal function.

Think of what dirt looks like when it's parched: hard, cracked, and wrinkled. The same thing happens to our bodies without enough water – it just takes longer and is harder to see. Except on our faces. It makes sense that since skin is 64% water, without proper hydration, our faces will become wrinkled and dull over time. Water is probably the cheapest anti-wrinkle, anti-aging potion available.

Lean tissue is made of more water than fat tissue. Since men naturally have more muscle due to the hormone testosterone, they are made of slightly more water than women. Women can even this out by lifting weights to increase muscle mass (which will have the added benefit of burning more calories).

How much water do we need? That really depends on your age, gender, activity level, diet and the climate, just to name a few.

I'm sure you're familiar with the adage to drink eight glasses of water a day. For most of us, that's easy to remember but harder to do. We do get water from our food – especially juicy fruits and non-starchy vegetables. Other beverages, like coffee, tea, juices and soda count to some degree, but your best bet is still water. Just plain water.

By the time we realize we're thirsty, we are already partially dehydrated. Too often we think we're hungry and we're just dehydrated. If you're craving a doughnut, drink a glass of water instead and see what happens.

Water – Good

Start your day with at least six ounces of hot water with the juice of half a lemon or lime. Drink this before you eat in the morning. It is a great way to wake up your digestive system. Another consideration for your digestion is drinking water with meals. It's okay to drink it before you start eating, but once you've taken your first bite, it is better not to drink anything. Drinking liquids during meals interferes with the digestive juices that are so critical to break down your food. If you must drink during a meal, only sip room temperature liquids (preferably water).

Always keep a glass of water on your desk and sip it throughout the day. Buy yourself a beautiful goblet or glass – something to make drinking water more of an experience. Buy a BPA-free container so you can keep water with you when you're out and about. Just be cautious about keeping water bottles in hot cars – that creates the perfect breeding ground for unhealthy germs.

Water – Better

BETTER than just drinking eight glasses of water a day, is to aim to drink half of your body weight in ounces. So, if you weigh 200 pounds, aim for 100 ounces, which coincidentally is approximately three liters; the daily amount recommended by the Mayo Clinic. Eight glasses are a good start, but in this example, drinking eight, eight ounce glasses for a total of 64 ounces of water, falls far short of the 100 ounces recommended by the Mayo Clinic.

To increase your water consumption, try adding four ounces every other day until you are at your optimal level. When you start increasing your water intake, you will need to pee more, it's true. But after a few days your body calms down and you will find your new normal, so stick with it. You can also just increase your amounts a lot slower.

As with food, it's better to stop drinking around 7:00 pm. It will allow your digestive juices to go to work and will decrease the likelihood of having to get up in the middle of the night to use the bathroom.

Drinking more water will naturally crowd out sugar-laden sodas and caffeine-laden coffee. Water is better for your waistline and easier on your budget.

Water – Best

In my house, we are definitely divided about the best source of water. Most men in my house were Boy Scouts who camped regularly and were willing to drink out of streams. I don't camp and I prefer filtered water. In many places tap water is perfectly safe. I will drink it when I need to, but when I fill my water bottle to have on my desk, it's filled with filtered water.

Most tap water contains chlorine to kill bacteria and microbes. In our water pipes that's a good thing but once that same chlorine enters our bodies, it continues to indiscriminately kill organisms. Some of what gets killed is needed by your body to keep other organisms in balance. I do my best to avoid chlorine – both inside and outside of my body. I have installed a chlorine filter on the shower head in my bathroom. My hair stylist immediately noticed the difference – she said my hair was a lot softer!

I've also noticed when I keep a bottle of water sitting on my desk, I can truly taste the difference between plain tap and filtered water. I've had clients tell me they just don't like the way water tastes. I always recommend they try again - with filtered water.

For the environment, I rarely drink bottled water. With awareness and planning, you can carry your own container and refill it. Most facilities now have water bottle filler stations in addition to traditional water fountains. Every little bit counts. If you must drink bottled water, please recycle.

At home or at work, keep a water filtration pitcher in your fridge or install a filter on one of your faucets. Both are simple solutions and far less expensive than drinking bottled water.

I prefer drinking out of glass, but plastic is okay as long as it is BPA-free. BPA stands for bisphenol A. which is an industrial chemical used to make some plastics and resins. Research has raised concerns that BPA can negatively affect our brains and cause additional issues in our children. While the studies are not conclusive, why take the risk? Be aware of the containers you use and the containers your food is in: packages that have the recycled numbers 3 & 7 probably contain BPA. Most canned foods are in cans lined with BPA resin. Look for food and beverage containers that are labeled "BPA free."

Water – Intentionally Simple

Find a pitcher and take the time to measure out what half your body weight in ounces looks like. It will be a great visual to understand how much water your body needs daily.

Next, commit to drinking that amount daily. (Again, ramp up slowly if you're not used to drinking a lot of water. Slow and steady wins the race.)

NOTES

STEP 5

Read Labels

Knowledge is power.
-Sir Francis Bacon

We're almost ready to start diving into food. But before we can do that, it's important to know what you're eating and the best way to do that is to read labels. Knowledge is power and reading labels will empower you to make informed choices. I just mentioned that most canned foods are lined with BPA. Those that aren't will clearly be labeled BPA-free. You just need to take the time to read the label before you buy.

I could easily fill the remainder of this book with label reading and what to look for. I encourage you to continue to learn on your own. Remember this book is a primer to get you started. With that in mind, I will help initiate you in the art of label-reading.

The first three ingredients listed on the label have the highest concentration. Often when a food is labeled "fat free" it means a whole lot of sugar was added to compensate for the missing fat. Fat free does not mean calorie free. Check the ingredients. If sugar, or one of its many pseudonyms (see below), is one of the first three ingredients, choose an alternative.

Other Names for Sugar
Source: Prevention Magazine and the USDA

Agave nectar
Anhydrous dextrose
Barley malt
Beet sugar
Blackstrap molasses
Brown rice syrup
Brown sugar
Buttered sugar
Cane juice crystals
Cane juice
Caramel
Carob syrup
Caster sugar
Coconut sugar
Confectioner's powdered sugar
Corn sweetener
Corn syrup
Corn syrup solids
Crystalline fructose
Date sugar
Demara sugar
Dextran
Dextrose
Diastatic malt
Diatase
Ethyl maltol
Evaporated cane juice
Fruit juice concentrates

Fructose
Galactose
Glucose
Golden sugar
Golden syrup
High-fructose corn syrup (HFCS)
Honey
Invert sugar
Lactose
Malt syrup
Maltodextrin
Maltose
Maple syrup
Molasses
Muscovado sugar
Nectars
Oat syrup
Organic raw sugar
Panela
Panocha
Raw sugar
Rice bran syrup
Rice syrup
Sorghum
Sorghum syrup
Sucrose
Sugar
Syrup

Tapioca syrup	White granulated sugar
Treacle	Yellow sugar
Turbinado sugar	

On the Nutrition Facts panel portion of the label, first look at the serving size. Most cans of soup, for instance, contain two servings. One serving size on a package of Oreos is three cookies (who can eat just three Oreos?) When you're aware of the serving size, you can more accurately review the rest of the label since each item listed is for one serving. The percentage of Daily Value (% DV) is based on 2000 calories a day. If you're trying to lose weight, you are probably eating less than 2000 calories and therefore the percentages listed would be higher for you.

The FDA allows food manufacturers to list an item containing 0.5 gms or less, of trans fat per serving as containing "0 gm" of trans fat. That may not sound like a lot, but if a bag of potato chips contains six servings and you eat the whole thing, you are really eating 3 grams of trans fat, even though the label would have you believe you aren't eating any trans-fat (0.5 gms per serving x 6 servings = 3 gms).

Trans fat is listed under the ingredients as hydrogenated oil or partially hydrogenated oil. So, if the food is labeled as containing "0 gm" of trans-fat, check the ingredients list to be sure. The American Heart Association recommends you limit your daily intake of trans-fat to less than two grams per day. Total avoidance is even better.

According to the American Heart Association, consuming trans-fat increases your bad cholesterol (LDL), while lowering your good cholesterol (HDL). It is also linked with higher incidences of heart disease, stroke and type 2 diabetes. Yikes!

Sugar is similarly treated: a product is allowed to be labeled "sugar free" when in reality it contains up to 0.5 gms of sugar. When you familiarize yourself with the different names for sugar, you will clearly see them listed in the ingredients list, even though the label says it's sugar free.

Read Labels – Good

Now that you know a little bit about what you're looking at when you read a food label, start choosing products with fewer ingredients - especially ingredients that are hard to pronounce. Things like Acetylated Monoglycerides, Dextrose and Color (red 40, yellows 5 & 6, blue 1). All are additives (these happen to be found in popular fruit-leather snacks, aimed at children) that bear little resemblance to real food. Some additives, like food coloring, have been linked to hyperactivity in children.

The FDA says the research is still inconclusive, but in Europe, the European Food Standards Agency was sufficiently convinced following the results of a study done in 2007 to ask manufacturers to voluntarily eliminate added artificial colors in food.

The first step in a GOOD practice is actually reading labels and choosing products with fewer ingredients.

Read Labels – Better

I believe one of the single most important steps you can take, starting today, is to eliminate foods containing high fructose corn syrup (HFCS).

According to Dr. Mark Hyman: "When used in moderation [high fructose corn syrup] is a major cause of heart disease, obesity, cancer, dementia, liver failure, tooth decay, and more." HFCS was created in the 1950's as a cheaper and sweeter alternative to sugar, but it wasn't widely used until the 1970's when it became a great solution for utilizing the bumper crop of corn.

Notice Dr. Hyman used the words "in moderation." Unfortunately, HFCS is rampant in our food. Candy and soda are obvious. But HFCS is also found in crackers, yogurt, salad dressings, ice cream, mac 'n cheese, canned fruit, soup, and so much more. It is actually challenging to find a loaf of bread without HFCS (or just plain corn syrup). It is so important to read labels!

Remember those two major hunger hormones: ghrelin and leptin? HFCS has been shown to reduce these hormones. So once again, you are likely to over-eat because HFCS have interfered with your body's innate ability to regulate your hunger. As a result, even though you eat and eat and eat, you never feel "full."

Canadian researchers have found that the brain lights up when consuming high fructose corn syrup the same way it does when snorting cocaine. Is it really just a coincidence that in the United States, obesity and the consumption of high fructose corn syrup have risen at the same time?

One study analyzed 43 countries and found that the prevalence of type 2 diabetes was higher in countries where HFCS was readily available.

Do your own research and see what makes sense to you. It's important to know what's in your food and it's important to know the source of your information.

Read Labels – Best

Eat mostly food that has no label – think whole foods: fruits, vegetables, lean meats. When you go grocery shopping, stay on the perimeter. Think of the way the typical grocery store is set up – most of the whole foods products are along the outside walls: produce, meat, dairy. Most of these foods have labels with the least ingredients, or even better, no labels at all. The closer you venture into the middle of the store, the more additives you will find listed on the packages of highly processed food.

Read Labels – Intentionally Simple

Take a moment right now and think of the five foods you eat most often (be sure to include salad dressing if that is a staple in your diet!) and write them down below. Next, commit to reading the labels of those five foods. The simplest way is to Google "Nutrition Facts [your food here]." Everything you want to know will pop up on your screen. Using what you have learned in this chapter, evaluate the ingredients – especially the first three listed.

Knowledge truly is power. With this new-found knowledge, you can make informed (and hopefully) healthier choices.

NOTES

Vegetables & Fruits

**Knowledge is knowing that a tomato is a fruit;
Wisdom is not putting it in a fruit salad.
-Miles Kington**

I purposely switched the order of the words because we are
bombarded, on a daily basis, with the mandate to EAT MORE
FRUITS AND VEGETABLES! My telling you to eat more fruits
and vegetables is not only redundant, but I am at risk of you tuning
me out. Of just being more noise. By saying vegetables and fruits,
maybe you'll read a little slower and actually digest (pun intended)
what I'm saying.

You already know you're supposed to eat more vegetables and fruits –
but why? The research and the studies in this area are vast and too
numerous to name here, but it's worth listing at least a few of the
benefits.

Initially, it was widely believed that eating more vegetables and
fruits would help ward off many types of cancers. Research has since

narrowed the thesis that certain vegetables (mainly the green, non-starchy variety) may protect against certain types of cancer (mouth, throat, stomach).

One of the most recent finds is that a diet rich in vegetables and fruits can lower your risk of cardiovascular disease and stroke. The World Health Organization lists cardiovascular disease as the number one cause of death worldwide. If you include cancer (the second highest cause of death), almost half of the deaths in the United States would fall into this group.

A fourteen year, Harvard-based study that followed 110,000 men and women showed that the more vegetables and fruits they consumed on an average daily basis, the lower their overall risk for developing cardiovascular disease.

A healthier gut is another benefit. There are two types of fiber: soluble and insoluble. Soluble fiber (found in, among other things, blueberries, cucumbers, and celery) dissolves in water and insoluble fiber (found in, among other things, apples, dark leafy vegetables, and broccoli), does not. Both fibers are important to your health.

Soluble fiber helps to slow down digestion to keep you feeling full longer. That may in turn help keep your blood sugar level more stable. Insoluble fiber will help food pass through your intestinal tract easier and prevent constipation. As you increase your fiber intake, it is important to drink enough water to help fiber do its job (see Step 4 – Water).

Vegetables & Fruits – Good

Before we get to how much is enough, start by honestly assessing how many vegetables and fruits you eat daily. A GOOD first Step is to just eat more than that. Even in the healthy circles I travel in, it's hard to find anyone who actually eats the recommended daily amount (that daily recommendation varies wildly depending on the source: anywhere from five to thirteen servings). How many servings did you eat yesterday? A GOOD Step is to just eat one more today.

What exactly constitutes a serving? 1/2 cup of vegetables or ½ cup of fruit is considered one serving. The exceptions are: one full cup of raw leafy greens like lettuce or spinach is one serving; ¼ cup of dried fruit is one serving; and a single (medium) sized piece of fruit, like an orange, apple, peach or pear, is considered one serving. To make it simple, for now, just consider ½ cup of a vegetable or fruit a serving. Aim to eat three - four cups.

If today you ate an apple, an orange, a salad made with 2 cups of leafy greens plus 1 cup of additional cut up vegetables (broccoli, scallions, cucumbers), and a few celery and carrot sticks, that would constitute six servings.

By eating more vegetables and fruits, you will naturally crowd out the junk. Remember the suggestion in Eating Basics (Step 2) to eat the apple before you eat the chocolate cake? I believe the more vegetables and fruits you eat, the less you'll want to eat the chocolate cake or the less of the chocolate cake you'll want to eat.

Vegetables & Fruits - Better

Now that you're eating more vegetables and fruits, pay attention to the kinds of vegetables and fruits you're eating. Familiarize yourself with the glycemic index (see next page). The Glycemic Index (GI) offers information on how different foods affect blood sugar and insulin. Generally, the lower a food is listed on the GI, the less it affects blood sugar and insulin levels. Less than 55 is considered low, while a value above 55 is considered high.

Why do we care about insulin? It's the hormone your body produces to keep your blood sugar level. When you eat foods high on the Glycemic Index, white bread, for example, your body pumps more and more insulin to counter-act the spike in your blood sugar. Eventually, the system breaks down and insulin can no longer do its job – that's called insulin resistant. Insulin resistance may lead to obesity and the potential for a wide range of chronic diseases.

Pay attention to where your fruit choices appear on the Glycemic Index. A good rule of thumb is the sweeter the fruit, the higher it is on the index. Bananas are routinely considered high/low or low/medium on the scale but the more they ripen, the sweeter they get and the higher they rank on the GI. Pasta is the same way – the more you cook it, the higher it rises on the GI. BETTER is to eat your bananas on the green side and your pasta *al dente*.

Speaking of pasta - also pay attention to serving size. The serving size for cooked pasta is around one cup. Measure it out at least one time to give yourself a visual example. Chances are you routinely eat more than one serving of pasta. Most restaurants will serve you several servings in a single meal because pasta is inexpensive, and they want you to feel like you're getting a good value.

It's important to pay attention to the serving size of fruit too – it's okay to eat a large slice of watermelon, but again, that might be the equivalent of several servings. That may equal your daily allowance for fruit, so, to round out the recommended servings, eat more vegetables.

FOOD	Glycemic Index
Apple	36
Banana	51
Cheerios	74
Date	42
Eggplant	15
Frosted Flakes	55
Grapefruit	25
Honey	61
Ice Cream, vanilla	60
Jelly Beans	80
Kiwi Fruit	52
Lentils	32
Macaroni and Cheese	64
Navy Beans	38
Orange	43
Popcorn	65
Quinoa	53
Raisins	64
Sweet Potato	54
Tomato	15
Udon Noodles	55
Vegetable Soup	48
Watermelon	76
Xoconostle	33
Yogurt, fruit	41
Zucchini	15

The Glycemic Index ranks foods from low (0) to high (100) where pure glucose (a.k.a. sugar) is 100. This chart is just an easy way to get you started by comparing a variety of (mostly) common carbohydrates from A – Z. The actual Glycemic Index number will vary according to the source, but this chart will give you a relative idea of how fast the carbs you're eating will increase your blood glucose levels.

Diabetics, who's bodies don't produce enough insulin to properly process blood sugar, fare better on a low glycemic diet. People trying to lose weight have an easier time of it on a low glycemic diet, whereas an athlete, after an intense workout, would want a high glycemic food to quickly replenish depleted blood sugar levels.

Vegetables & Fruits - Best

Eat more green leafy vegetables and save fruit for an afternoon snack. In Eating Basics (Step 2), I suggested you eat your sugar indulgence before 3:00 p.m. Although you may not consider fruit an "indulgence," it would also fit in this category. Fruit has sugar in it and while the natural fructose in an apple is still far better than the potentially hormone-altering sugar in high fructose corn syrup, too much sugar will still throw your body out of balance. That's also why this Step is called vegetables and fruits – to put the emphasis on vegetables.

Here are a few easy ideas for incorporating healthier vegetables into your daily diet: exchange your iceberg lettuce with the more nutrient dense romaine lettuce; eat sweet potatoes instead of the plain white variety and add grated carrots to pasta sauce. The next time you go grocery shopping, buy a vegetable you don't normally eat. Corn, green beans, and white potatoes are starchy vegetables and best eaten sparingly. Learn your greens: kale, spinach and Swiss chard. I mastered the art of roasting kale – you can find the simple step-by-step recipe on my website: www.mairhill.com.

Build bigger, better salads. Since we're talking about BEST practices and eating lots of leafy greens, I want to caution you about salad dressings. This is where you really need to read labels, or better yet, learn to make your own. When you slather rich, creamy, sugar-laden dressings on all those beautiful leafy greens, you are adding unnecessary fat, sugar, and empty calories to an otherwise perfectly healthy choice.

Make a simple dressing with extra virgin olive oil (EVOO), a squeeze of lemon juice and a few dried herbs (I like an Italian herb mix, no salt added). Use that as a base to start and experiment with other additions.

Beware of pesticides on your vegetables and fruits. Every year the Environmental Working Group (EWG) publishes a list called the Dirty Dozen™. It ranks, in order, the vegetables and fruits that are grown using the most pesticides. They also publish a list called The Clean Fifteen™ which lists the least contaminated. The complete list actually is a lot longer than just the Dirty Dozen™ (to see the entire list, visit the EWG website: www.ewg.org). An example of both lists is included on the next page.

Dirty Dozen™	**Clean Fifteen™**
Strawberries	Avocados
Spinach	Sweet Corn
Kale	Pineapples
Nectarines	Sweet Peas - Frozen
Apples	Onions
Grapes	Papayas
Peaches	Eggplants
Cherries	Asparagus
Pears	Kiwis
Tomatoes	Cabbages
Celery	Cauliflower
Potatoes	Cantalope
	Broccoli
	Mushrooms
	Honeydew

Use this list to determine when it pays to buy organic. For example, apples are traditionally on top of the Dirty Dozen™ list so buying organic is the BEST choice. Avocados, on the other hand, top the Clean Fifteen™ list for least contaminated so organic isn't necessary. This list is updated annually so for the latest information, please visit the EWG website (www.ewg.org). EWG is a not-for-profit group and for a small donation, they will send you the EWG's Shopper's Guide to Pesticides in Produce.

Another way to reduce the pesticide residue is to wash your vegetables and fruits well. To wash apples, I fill a spray bottle with 1/3 apple cider vinegar and 2/3 filtered water and spray each apple before I wash it. When I have time, I soak my vegetables and fruits in a mixture of 2 TB apple cider vinegar per gallon of water. When I have even more time, I use the method discovered and perfected by Dr. Parcells.

Dr. Parcells was the head of the Nutrition Department at Sierra States University and in the 1960's she discovered that when she used a Clorox bath to cleanse her foods, not only was the taste of the food improved, but it extended the storage life by at least two weeks. She experimented with all kinds of bleach and determined that to be effective, it had to be Clorox bleach. I first read about Dr. Parcells in *The Fat Flush Plan* by Dr. Ann Louise Gittleman.

I have regularly used the Clorox bath to clean my vegetables and fruits. It's true, the vegetables and fruits do stay fresher longer and there is no Clorox taste.

To make your own Clorox bath, start with one gallon of filtered water. Add one teaspoon (per gallon) of Clorox bleach. Vegetables and fruits (with the exception of leafy greens), can be soaked for thirty minutes. Leafy greens can be soaked for fifteen minutes. After this initial soaking time, remove the vegetables and fruits and place them in another bowl of clean, filtered water. Soak for an additional ten minutes then rinse and dry thoroughly before storing in the refrigerator.

Vegetables And Fruits – Intentionally Simple

Add a vegetable to each one of your meals. At first, maybe that just means eating a carrot with your cereal, but as you get more creative, you'll learn to add shredded carrots to your pasta sauce, or sauté some spinach with your scrambled eggs, or keep cut up broccoli in your fridge to eat with hummus as a nice side to your lunch.

Think of fruit as a dessert and eat it sparingly.

NOTES

STEP 7

Protein

Man's health and well-being depends upon...the proper functioning of the myriad proteins that participate in the intricate synergisms of living systems.
- Stanford Moore

Every cell in your body contains protein. It is necessary to help your cells repair and restore themselves. It's also important for keeping your blood sugar level. Remember, level blood sugar is important, so your body isn't dumping excess insulin into your blood stream. The type of protein and the amounts your body needs really vary by individual. I was a pescatarian for three years which means I ate fish, but no other animal protein. I found that my body just works better when I eat animal protein.

Too often I will have a client announce they plan to become a vegetarian for no other reason than they believe it will just be healthier. Fundamentally I agree that a plant-based diet rich in whole foods will do wonders for your body, but this is something you need to experiment with for yourself. And of course, check with your doctor first.

Begin with "Meatless Mondays" and then maybe add a second meatless day during the week. If you start slowly, it will be easier to learn the proper way to incorporate a vegetarian diet into your lifestyle. It requires education and dedication. It's too easy to substitute the all-beef hamburger for French fries, pasta and bread and fool yourself that you're going to get healthier by not eating meat.

Amino acids combine to form proteins and together they are the building blocks of life. Your body does not make them naturally, so you need to get them from your food. Complete proteins contain all nine essential amino acids. Meat and eggs are two examples of complete proteins. Plant sources are incomplete protein, but when combined (think whole grains and beans), they form a complete protein. It is not required to eat them together to reap the benefits, just be sure they are eaten in the same day. The combination of rice and beans is a popular choice for a complete protein.

How much is enough? Again, the range varies wildly depending on the source and your own personal lifestyle. Pregnant/nursing women, athletes and people trying to lose weight, all need more protein. For the rest of us, a good daily average is 46 grams for women and 56 grams for men. A 3-ounce serving of protein is about the size of a deck of cards, or the palm of your hand, and contains about 21 grams of protein.

Protein - Good

It's a GOOD practice to include protein as part of your breakfast (within an hour of waking up and after you've had your lemon water): Greek yogurt; turkey bacon (it's really good if you have the time to bake it); a smoothie with protein powder; leftovers from dinner the night before or two eggs are just a few suggestions.

If you're using protein powder be sure to read the label. Just because it's sold in a vitamin store doesn't make it good for you. If you plan to make protein powder a regular source of your protein, it's worth taking the time to research healthier and more pure powders. There are a lot of good resources on-line. I prefer vegetarian protein powders containing pea, hemp or rice protein, instead of the traditional whey protein (which contains dairy).

Think outside the box! There is no rule saying you must eat breakfast foods for breakfast. In fact, most cereals are sugar-laden, carb-heavy, empty calorie loaded foods that will spike your blood sugar level and leave you tired and hungry. Eat your leftover dinner – especially if it contained lean meat.

Eggs are another great choice. It seems over the years the egg has been our friend and our enemy. I'm not sure which it is at the moment. The fact is, eggs are a complete protein – that means they contain all the amino acids your body needs. But to reap the full benefit of eating an egg, you need to eat the whole thing. Roughly half of the protein is found in the yolk. And yes, the yolk has cholesterol but your body needs cholesterol to function. When you don't get enough cholesterol, your liver compensates by producing more of it – if you eat more cholesterol, your liver just produces less.

Your body prefers to be in balance and when you feed it properly, it automatically works toward that balance. The best eggs are Omega 3 enriched and are from pasture raised chickens. There are studies showing it is safe to eat three whole eggs a day. I'm not suggesting you do; I am saying you don't need to be afraid of eggs.

Rotate. Mix it up. Plan your week on Sunday evening and know when you'll have time to cook eggs in the morning and when grabbing a smoothie will be a faster choice.

Hard boil six eggs and just keep them in the refrigerator for a quick snack or a protein addition to one of your meals.

Protein - Better

Include a protein source at every meal. When you spread it out during the day, you continue to keep your blood sugar level which will help cut your cravings for junk, among other benefits.

Quinoa is an excellent source of protein. Often labeled as a grain, quinoa is actually a seed. Like eggs, because it contains all nine essential amino acids, it is considered a complete protein.

Even before the Incas (1200 – 1400 AD), the Andean people (3200 BC) haled quinoa as one of their main food sources. In other words, quinoa has been around for a very long time. The United Nations General Assembly declared 2013 "The International Year of Quinoa" to acknowledge the ancestral practices of the Andean people which enabled quinoa to still be available today.

Cooking directions are similar to rice: ½ cup of quinoa to 1 cup of water, bring to a boil, lower heat, cover, cook for 20 minutes. When it's done, remove the pan from the heat, place a paper towel between the lid and the pot to absorb extra moisture. After ten minutes, fluff with a fork and serve. Quinoa is great cold and easily frozen for eating later.

Quinoa has an outer coating that can turn bitter, so before cooking, it's a good idea to rinse it to remove this coating. Quinoa is good hot or cold. It's easy to transport.

For a simple, delicious, nutritious and healthy lunch, add half an avocado and a splash of Bragg's Liquid Amino Acids (a good substitute for soy sauce – no MSG) to one cup of cooked quinoa.

Nuts are a decent source of protein but because they are loaded with fat, albeit healthy fat, you need to eat them sparingly. For instance, approximately 23 almonds are considered one serving. Raw nuts are certainly healthier than dry roasted. If you buy them in bulk, you can keep them in the refrigerator to keep them fresh. I like to keep them in glass jars. Nuts also freeze well.

Explore the alternatives to peanut butter – there are many delicious nut – and seed - butters available including almond butter and sunflower seed butter. For any of the nut butters, try to buy those that have the oil at the top. Read the label – those butters typically only have the nut and maybe salt in the jar.

BETTER is to buy these natural nut butters and stir them yourself. After you've stirred the nut butter and mixed the oil in thoroughly, store them in the refrigerator upside down. The nut butter will be the perfect consistency when you want to spread it on your bread (or carrot stick). Again, use sparingly. A serving size of nut butter is usually only two tablespoons.

The nut butters that don't require stirring will include unnecessary added ingredients like palm oil to keep the nut butter from separating.

Protein - Best

Once you're eating more protein, and spreading it throughout the day, it's time to be aware of your protein source. Organic, or at least free range, grass fed, is better than most commercial meat. Do your best to avoid deli meats. Some are restructured meat products and are formed from binding together smaller chunks. All kinds of chemicals – including possibly nitrites – are added in that process.

Like the pesticides on our vegetables and fruits, our meat supply is tainted with hormones such as synthetic estrogens and testosterone. Recombinant bovine growth hormone, or rBGH, is another controversial hormone that increases the amount of milk dairy cows produce and winds up in our dairy supply.

Know your source. Ask your butcher or the person behind the meat counter where they get their meat. Organic is BEST. Even Costco and Wal-Mart have made more organic choices available. If organic is not an option, limit the number of hormones and other additives that are often added to meat. Learn to eat rice and beans, quinoa or eggs for alternative protein sources.

Fish is also a great source of protein. Like the Dirty Dozen™ list that's published for vegetables and fruits, the Environmental Defense Fund (EDF) rates fish for a variety of health factors including sustainability, mercury levels (or other hormones), and lists them in a range from Eco-friendly to Eco-Worst.

Farm-raised fish are likely to be fed hormone additives the same way domestic cattle are. When buying farm-raised fish, ask if they were organically farmed in an enclosed tank or pond or were they farmed in a polluted ocean?

Be sure your source is reputable. High-end fish such as salmon, red snapper and grouper have all been involved in fish fraud: tilapia was sold as red snapper; farm-raised salmon was sold as wild caught – and customers paid accordingly. Wild Alaska salmon is only available fresh in the spring so if you're buying wild Alaska salmon in December and it's marked "fresh," it's likely been frozen. In the United States, Atlantic salmon is all farm-raised. If you eat tuna from a can, read the label and be sure it's packed in water instead of calorie-laden oil.

Lean meats, like chicken and turkey, are better than red meat. And by chicken, I don't mean hot wings! Eat pork very sparingly. (If you're interested in knowing more, read an article titled "6 Horrifying Things about Pork Everyone Should Know" by Martha Rosenberg. The title pretty much says it all.)

To reduce fat and calories, broil or bake your meats instead of frying. Grilling is good as long as you don't burn the meat. The black char is often considered to be carcinogenic. Also, remove the skin before eating. You can cook it with the skin on to prevent the meat from drying out, but the skin has a disproportionate amount of unwanted fat and calories.

Protein – Intentionally Simple

Add quinoa to your dict as a protein source.

It freezes well, so make a big batch at the start of your week and freeze it in ½ cup servings. Add it to your salad or your soup. It's an easy and healthy way to increase your protein consumption.

NOTES

STEP 8

Prepping/Shopping

By failing to prepare you are preparing to fail.
-Benjamin Franklin

Remember, this book is a primer – a way to get you started on your own GOOD PLAN to a healthier lifestyle. For that reason, I limited the food portion to vegetables and fruits and protein. If you build 80% of your diet around these categories and eliminate high fructose corn syrup from the other 20%, you will be well on your way to better health. When you focus on these whole foods, there will be less room for all the processed foods you might currently be eating. Those are the foods that have long, unpronounceable ingredients listed on the label, are laden with unwanted fat and calories, and probably rank high on the Glycemic Index.

In order to further help you create your own GOOD PLAN from these pages, you will need to incorporate them into your everyday life. I believe a GOOD PLAN is a real-life plan. One you can actually do.

I refer to Step 1 – Mindset. What do you want? And what are you willing to do? This isn't about going from zero to sixty overnight, it's about taking one, ONE! idea that you've read so far and trying it on. Does it fit? Does it need a little alteration? What would make it better? Determine if it makes sense for you to make it part of your routine. It will take desire, discipline, prepping and planning to make your life a healthier one. It's never too late to start!

The older I get, the more I appreciate that I've (mostly) always taken good care of myself. Our bodies are amazing! And very forgiving! Once you begin to treat your body better, it will respond accordingly. Once you start to feel the difference, you will never want to go back to the way you were feeling.

Prepping/Shopping - Good

Plan tomorrow before today ends. Use what you already have in the house and figure out what you will eat for each of your meals and your snacks using what you've learned in the first seven Steps. Keep it very simple. It's so much easier to stay on track when you know what you're going to eat next and it's already waiting for you. If you can make your whole lunch before you go to bed and keep it in the fridge, even better. You will have a calmer morning. You will have time to eat breakfast.

Start making a list of things you would like to have – like lemons, quinoa or romaine lettuce. That way, your shopping list will be ready when you have time to shop. Shopping with a list will also save you money by helping you avoid impulse buys. Grocery stores are designed to tempt you to buy impulsively. Be aware the next time you are shopping. Look around. It's no accident that items such as candy bars and soda – are near the registers. Stick with the items on your list.

Prepping/Shopping - Better

Make time over the weekend to plan a week's worth of meals. You don't even have to do this on your own. There are countless books and websites to help you with this. Apps too. Whether you want something basic, or Paleo, or vegetarian, someone has already figured it out for you. Make your list and shop for it. There are apps to help you keep track of this too.

You will begin to build your own data base of favorite recipes and meals. If you have kids, let them help too. Agree to try at least one new recipe and/or food every week. Be adventurous. Make sure all the colors of the rainbow are represented in your food at some point during the week.

According to researchers at the Washington Center for Obesity, most Americans routinely eat no more than 30 different foods and they take about four days to cycle through all of them. Commit to expanding the number of different foods you eat.

How many do you eat? Take a few minutes and write down what you can remember eating over the past few days. Is it more or less than thirty?

As you go through your week, be aware of what works and what needs some tweaking. Remember this is real-life – not just something you're trying for a few days. Incorporating these Steps is a practice - a journey to a healthier you.

Prepping/Shopping - Best

Prep most of your food yourself. It will be healthier, less expensive, and you will be more connected to the food you are eating. When you rely less on convenience foods, even prepackaged vegetables, you are eliminating added chemicals and sodium from your diet.

Plan to prep. I try to shop on the same two days every week. Then I know when I get home, I will spend about ninety minutes washing, drying and prepping what I bought. Or, hire a local teenager to do this for you. When you're done, you'll have a refrigerator full of clean, healthy vegetables and fruits and they stay fresher longer.

I always prep several heads of romaine lettuce, a bunch or two of kale and a bunch of spinach. These greens are the basis for the salads we eat most nights with dinner. I also cut up and store red peppers, celery, carrots, scallions, broccoli, and cauliflower. I only cut up cucumbers just before I use them. Remember serving sizes? A salad made with all these vegetables can easily count for three of your recommended daily servings.

You can do the same with boneless, skinless chicken breasts. Bake 3-4 at a time with a little bar-be-cue sauce (read the label – no HFCS!) or a little olive oil and garlic salt. Bake at 350 degrees and check after 20 minutes. Invest in a meat thermometer so you know your meat is cooked properly. You will save yourself a lot of money and eat much more nutritionally than buying fast food.

Keep a running grocery list. Schedule your grocery shopping the same way you would any appointment. Never shop hungry – you are more likely to buy junk food – and overspend. Shop the perimeter of the grocery store. Eat whole, fresh vegetables. Pay attention to the Dirty Dozen™ and Clean Fifteen™ lists.

Fresh is better than frozen and frozen is better than canned.

Prepping/Shopping - Intentionally Simple

Ask a friend for her favorite vegetable recipe – or go on-line to find a new one of your own. Just Google "Best [insert vegetable here] recipe."

Whether you're adventurous and willing to try something you've never even thought about before (Celeriac? Fennel? Bok Choy?) or just want a new way to cook your old standby (Carrots? Peas? Onions?), take a few minutes now to find the recipe and schedule it into your week.

NOTES

STEP 9

Exercise

You can't out exercise a bad diet.
-Dr. Mark Hyman

Even though what you eat is more important than exercising to improve your overall health, A GOOD PLAN must include exercise. Moving your body will keep your joints lubricated and fluid. The easier your joints move, the more likely you are to exercise. Being physically active is crucial for the health of your heart, your lungs, and your brain and that's just the beginning.

If weight loss is your goal, it doesn't really matter how long you exercise if you continue to eat potato chips and other processed junk food. Nonetheless, moving your body has its own benefits and rewards like improved strength, stamina, mobility, mood, and sleep: all benefits needed to live and enjoy your life to the fullest.

Exercise has been shown to make you smarter. After a cardio workout, your brain is busy making new brain cells, new connections to help you learn. In one study, if the cardio workout required participants to think, like tennis or Zumba, they were even more likely to succeed at complicated tasks post exercise.

Exercise will improve your mood. "Runner's High" is real. During exercise, your body releases the feel-good brain chemicals like serotonin, dopamine, and norepinephrine. These chemicals have also been shown to lower stress – they almost mimic the effects of anti-depressants - without the side effects. Exercising will help you appreciate your body and may, therefore, boost your overall confidence.

Find an exercise buddy. When someone else is counting on you to show up, it will give you that extra boost to get out of bed or rearrange your schedule in order to honor that commitment. Mutual support will help both of you stay accountable and help you to get back on track if you fall off. Most importantly, an exercise buddy will make your workouts fun and it will be easier to try something new: if you've always wanted to take a Zumba class, but didn't want to show up alone, there's safety in numbers. Shared experiences – like trying something new together – will deepen your connection and keep you motivated.

Walking is certainly the easiest place to start. It's free. You can do it anywhere, for any length of time, and at any pace. Committing to a walking routine may inspire you to make healthier choices in other areas of your life, including the food you eat.

Whether you walk a mile or run a mile, you burn approximately 100 calories - the same number of calories contained in a medium apple. Obviously, if you're running, you can cover more miles in less time than walking the same distance.

It is often cited that to benefit from a walking program you need to walk "briskly" for 150 – 300 minutes per week. "Brisk" is considered at least 100 steps per minute. It's easy to measure while walking on a treadmill.

Walking daily and drinking the BEST amount of water will help eliminate constipation issues. It really is that easy, but it won't be instant. Be patient with your body. You didn't get to the condition you're in overnight, give your body time to adjust and heal with your new, healthier habits.

When you create an exercise program, start slowly. If you've been sedentary for a while, or have other medical conditions, please consult your doctor. A GOOD PLAN is one you can do. So instead of starting at sedentary and expecting yourself to become a true gym rat in a matter of days, follow the Steps below and increase the levels of your workouts according to what your body is telling you. The most important thing is to just start.

Exercise – Good

Move your body. Dance around the house. Swim in the pool. Jump on a rebounder. Just move your body. Every day. Walking is a very GOOD place to start. Buy a Fitbit, a simple pedometer, or other tracking device and aim for 10,000 steps every day.

You don't even have to go outside, although the fresh air is a bonus. Most indoor malls have a walking program and are open early to accommodate walkers before the stores open. Check online for the nearest walking trails.

Any excuse you can find during your day matters. At work; take the stairs instead of the elevator, park in the very last parking spot, walk to talk to a co-worker instead of emailing, and take the long way to the bathroom. At home; march in place during television commercials and when you're out, park your car once and walk around town to do errands. At the very least, dedicate at least ten minutes every day to walk.

Exercise – Better

Break a sweat every day, or at least most days. This means you are exercising at a faster pace and working your heart even BETTER. Remember your heart is a muscle so it can be conditioned just like the biceps on your arms. Both will get stronger when exercised properly.

Aim for at least thirty minutes every day. You can break this up into two 15-minute sessions or three 10-minute sessions.

Even BETTER is to find an exercise you like. There is something for everyone; from Aerobics to Zumba. Experiment. You don't need to join a gym – chances are your local community center offers affordable classes. Ask around. Be open. Check out YouTube or the website of your favorite exercise guru for free content. (The internet is filled with free exercise options, however, as with anything, know your source. Just because it's on the internet – and free – doesn't make it safe.)

Exercise – Best

Add resistance training to your regimen. Cardio is a great start, but to make significant changes to your body, you need to add resistance training. You don't even have to lift traditional weights; your own body weight is perfect. Push-ups, squats, lunges, and pull-ups all use nothing more than your own weight to build muscle. Exercise bands are another alternative.

Again, you can find a lot of free routines on-line, join a class or pair up with a buddy and just make it up as you go along. Fifteen minutes, two to three times a week will make a big difference. Remember I mentioned Jorge Cruise? Check out his book called *8 Minutes in the Morning* for a very simple way to get started with resistance training. Or Google "fast whole body workout."

Lean muscle burns more calories than fat. As you get more and more into an exercise routine, it's easy to justify eating more because you've "earned it" or you already burned off all those calories so it's "okay." Don't fall into that trap. It takes more effort and longer than you think to burn off one hundred calories (remember walking one mile will burn off the calories contained in the aforementioned medium apple but at three hundred calories, the typical glazed doughnut will require three miles!)

It's even more important to fuel your body properly when you exercise. It's important before you exercise so you have the energy to sustain your workout and it is important post-workout because that's when your body begins to repair the muscles you used. It's in this repair process that your muscles get stronger.

And ladies, it is a fallacy that lifting weights will make you bulky. You'd have to lift heavy weights over a long period of time and really trim most of the fat off your body for your muscles to show. We are just not built that way.

As we age, our muscle mass decreases. By the time we're 50, we've lost almost 10%. Think of what you do in your everyday life: lift children, (maybe grandchildren), carry groceries, climb stairs, etc. It's important to build and maintain lean muscles for us to live life to our fullest potential.

If you'd like to lift weights and do cardio exercise in the same session, start with the weights. You'll able to lift longer if you're not fatigued first from a cardio workout.

Taking care of our bodies will enable us to physically do what we want to do, when we want to do it, for as long as possible.

Exercise – Intentionally Simple

Find a treadmill and adjust your pace until you're walking 100 steps per minute. Feel what that "brisk" walk feels like.

Next, make a date to go for a walk. Whether it's with a friend, your partner, your child or a co-worker, look at your schedule and set aside twenty minutes to go for a walk. Write it in your calendar – treat it like an appointment – it is that important. Knowing someone will be waiting for you (and counting on you!) will encourage you to keep your date.

Set out your clothes the night before or remember to bring your walking shoes (and socks) to work with you. Do whatever you need to do to keep your walking date.

NOTES

STEP 10

Happiness

Gratefulness is a practice, just like happiness is a choice. -Russell Simmons

Happiness is a choice – you get to make it every day. Positive Psychology is the scientific study of what makes a good life. I'm not sure we actually need science to tell us, although science has proven it is better to give than to receive. Several studies show that when participants were given money and told they could spend it on themselves or on someone else, those who spent it on someone else reported feeling happier. The same is true in a study that looked at who was happier: the person giving support or the person receiving the support. The majority of those lending support reported being happier.

A woman named Hannah Brencher launched a project called *The World Needs More Love Letters* in her senior year of college. She wrote several dozen love letters and left them all over campus. It caught on and soon other college students were doing it on their own campuses. It spread from there. People started finding love letters tucked between books, amid cereal boxes on grocery store shelves, left on the bus seat next to them. They were addressed simply to YOU.

The writers of these anonymous letters benefit as much, if not more than the recipients. The letters always seem to find the right person. Proof that something so simple, can prove to be so powerful. You can read more at www.moreloveletters.com

Stress, on the other hand, is a huge buzz kill. It's the complete opposite of happiness. It is very hard to be happy when you're stressed. The opposite is true too: it's hard to be stressed when you're happy.

When you're stressed, your body produces cortisol. It's the hormone that helps your body create instant energy because stress tells your body danger is coming and prepares you to flee (fight or flight syndrome). Cortisol, like insulin, promotes the production of fat. Since your belly has lots of cortisol receptors, this is where the fat is drawn and where it stays.

Belly fat is a fairly accurate predictor of your health. A big belly nearly doubles your risk of dying prematurely. The Body Mass Index (BMI) for determining obesity became popular in the 1980's. There are plenty of websites which enable you to plug in your individual numbers and see you where you fall on the range from underweight to obese. Because it uses a height-weight ratio, it fails to differentiate between fat and muscle and therefore provides an incomplete picture: someone who is very muscular could actually be considered obese using the BMI method.

Use BMI as one tool in your toolbox to assess your overall (relative) health. As you get fitter, your BMI will decrease.

Something far easier, and perhaps a more accurate predictor of obesity, is the relationship between your waist size and your height. Ideally your waist is half the size of your height. So, if you are six feet tall, which is 72," then 36" is the ideal waist size for you. Obviously less than 36" is good too.

If, however, your waist is 36" and you are NOT six feet tall, you really need to start making healthier choices. Measure your belly above your hips and below your rib cage. You can suck it in as best you can - it's not cheating because the dangerous belly fat is deep inside.

In really, really simple terms, being less stressed means less cortisol means less belly fat means a longer life. Less stress, more happiness. One doesn't automatically mean the other, but what if you work on both of them?

Happiness - Good

Make your bed every day. No kidding. It's on almost every "How to be Happier" list I've read. I don't know if it's because you've slowed down enough to take the time to make it or if it's the feel good feelings that come over you when you see a nicely made bed, or simply the sense of having accomplished something so early in the day, but it doesn't get much simpler than that. Just make your bed every day.

Why stop at simply making your bed? A cluttered desk, a cluttered closet, a cluttered environment leads to a cluttered mind. Clearing clutter is an industry all by itself and certainly beyond the scope of this book.

Marie Kondo took clutter clearing to a new level by inspiring people to keep only possessions which "spark joy."

Another GOOD place to start is with one of my favorite books on the subject: *Creating Sacred Space with Feng Shui* by Karen Kingston. It's full of practical advice, especially if you feel like a slave to all of your stuff.

Clearing your clutter can be as simple as committing to putting things away when you are finished using them or setting aside ten minutes every night before you go to bed to tidy your living space. When you pick up a pen that's out of ink, instead of putting it back in the drawer, throw it away. Now.

Have a place for everything and keep everything in its place. Resist the urge to buy more than will fit in that drawer or closet (the store will be happy to hold the extra inventory for you). Perhaps adopt a "net zero" policy – otherwise known as one-in-one-out. If you buy a new pair of shoes, make a deal with yourself that you will donate one currently residing in your closet.

Make a list of what Thomas J. Leonard calls "tolerations;" those areas of your home such as that drawer with the dried out pen, that closet that is so full it doesn't close properly or a dining room table that is so full you can't remember the last time you served a meal on it. Plan to tackle one item on your list per week or per month until they are all gone. Any time you walk into a room or open a closet and it's cluttered, it's an immediate energy drain – and one that can be easily eliminated.

Happiness - Better

As you've worked your way through the first nine Steps, you've been getting better and better at making yourself and your health a priority. Mental health is important too. Now it's time to explore what makes you happy and do more of it. Commit to it. Thirty minutes a day of "me" time. What does that look like? What do you like to do?

Imagine setting aside thirty minutes a day just for you. Does that seem impossible? Does your life already feel too full to find thirty more minutes to do something fun? (I promise you it's not too full AND the rest of your day will be easier because you spent these thirty minutes on yourself.)

Before you dismiss this idea entirely (because you tend to live in the land of overwhelm), maybe in the beginning, you schedule that thirty minutes just one time this week and you add thirty minutes each week until you're doing it every day. Schedule it. Write it in your planner. Protect it. Honor it. Thirty minutes, just for you.

Maybe this week you just sit and ponder what wonderful things you would do with that gift (to yourself) of thirty minutes: read a book; take a bath; learn a new language; learn to play an instrument; start that photo project that's been on the back burner forever; learn to knit; learn to Salsa; learn to cook. Use your imagination – your choices are limitless.

Maybe it would be a different activity every day of the week or you would just rotate through a few of them. Maybe it would be an activity of the month. Again, the possibilities are endless! (These thirty minutes does not include prepping/shopping, exercising or any of the other Steps in this book – unless it's to experiment with new, healthier recipes.)

The first action in this process is to decide to do it. To allow yourself time to think about it and get excited about it – remember this is something fun! Something you want to do! Not merely another item on your TO DO list that will cause you angst and anxiety until you "get it done."

Start simply. Set a timer – literally for thirty minutes – and at the end of thirty minutes, stop. Know that you get to do it again tomorrow. If you are as starved as most people are, for pure, unadulterated "me" time, it will be too easy to lose yourself in that book or class or project. Before you know it, three hours have passed and things that might have needed to get done fall by the wayside. Now you've just caused yourself a new source of stress because you're behind. All because you allowed yourself thirty minutes but took three hours. Set yourself up to win. Set a timer and honor your commitment to yourself: thirty minutes every day.

Happiness – Best

Since we started with Mindfulness in Step 1, it's fitting that we come full circle and end the same way. This time, instead of using your mind to be aware, the BEST practice in Step 10 for Happiness is to let your mind be free. Empty. Devoid of thought.

Develop a meditation practice. Start slowly. Just follow your breath.

Dr. Andrew Weil promotes what he calls 4-7-8 breathing. Very simply, let your tongue rest on the roof of your mouth behind your front teeth. Exhale completely through your mouth. Now you are ready to begin. Close your mouth and inhale through your nose for a count of 4. Hold your breath for a count of 7. Exhale slowly, through your mouth for a count of 8. Repeat this whole cycle 4 times (after one month, work up to 8 repetitions, max). Repeat this whole process at least two times daily.

It will take practice to inhale sufficient breath quickly enough in the first four counts to enable you to exhale that same breath slowly to the count of eight. You can easily find demonstrations of this technique on YouTube or on my website: www.mairhill.com.

The benefits of the 4-7-8 breathing technique really come after 4-6 weeks. According to Dr. Weil, 4-7-8 breathing will slow your heart rate, lower your blood pressure and improve your digestion. Use it to cut cravings for junk food or before you react negatively to someone cutting you off in traffic or fight with a co-worker. If you get up in the middle of the night, when you get back into bed, use this technique to fall asleep again.

You can also begin your meditation practice by daydreaming. Five minutes every day. Just close your eyes and let your imagination loose. What would you do with $1,000.000.00? $100,000,000.00? Imagine living on a tropical island. Maybe you've always dreamed of being a rock star – imagine yourself singing to a packed stadium. This is designed to be fun! If the thoughts you start thinking don't feel good, choose another scenario.

You can even do this sitting at your desk. If your work environment doesn't lend itself to five uninterrupted minutes, what about in your car? Think outside your cubicle. Again, set a timer. Five minutes. You get to do it again tomorrow.

Even if you never move beyond 4-7-8 breathing or five minutes of daydreaming, if you do it daily, you will reap benefits. Ideally, this practice will just leave you hungry for more. More time to empty your mind. More time to meditate.

Meditation is meant to be simple. Either sit up straight in a chair or lie down (you want your spine straight). If you're prone to falling asleep (that's actually a sign you have a sleep debt that needs to be paid), it's better to sit in a chair. Feet flat on the floor, back straight. Be comfortable. Close your eyes and just follow your breath. When random thoughts start flooding in, look at them like you would look at a helium-filled balloon and let them go. Watch them float away and go back to your breath. Repeat.

There are hundreds of books and recordings available on meditation, so they obviously go into a lot more detail than I do here. I just want to show you it really is that simple to get started.

Meditation is actually energizing so it is BEST to practice in the morning instead of before you go to sleep. Midday is a great option too. Just start. Use a timer. Start with five minutes and work your way up to twenty minutes. Every day.

Because it is a practice – the more you do it, the easier it will get. If you can meditate in the same spot at roughly the same time every day, that will make it even easier. Your body will know what to do when you sit down in that space. The important thing is to just start in whatever manner fits your lifestyle now. Remember, a GOOD PLAN is one you can do.

Meditation will make you calmer in your daily interactions. It will take more to get you rattled and upset. Clearing your mind allows more to flow into it. Your creativity will increase. Your productivity will increase. Your happiness will increase.

Shawn Achor does a TED Talk (www.ted.com) called "The Happy Secret to Better Work." It is twelve very worthwhile minutes. In it he explains why we have it all backwards. We are brought up to believe that if we just work hard enough, we will be successful and once we're successful, we'll be happy. He continues by pointing out that most of us, once we reach what we consider success, just raise the bar. So, if we think we have to achieve a certain goal to be successful and happiness is always on the other side, once we raise the bar again, happiness remains out of reach.

We need to retrain our brains to accept happiness now, just as we are, with what we have. Shawn calls it the Happiness Advantage (and he wrote a book by the same name) because when you are happy, your brain releases dopamine. Dopamine makes you feel good, and it turns on all the learning centers in your brain which make you more creative and more productive. An added benefit for you sales people – turning on these learning centers in your brain will even make you a better sales person!

Happiness, like most things in life, is a choice. You can choose to be happy now and your success will surely follow.

Happiness – Intentionally Simple

Next time you talk to someone on the telephone, whether it's for work or pleasure, and regardless of who initiated the call, before you even say hello, SMILE.

Obviously, the person on the other end of the line can't physically see you and that smile on your face, but they will be able to hear that smile in your voice.

Have you ever watched someone texting – and they're sitting there smiling? You can't help but smile with them, even though you have no idea what's making them so happy. It's the same principal. Your smile will be the good kind of infectious.

NOTES

CONCLUSION

Woohooo! I am so proud of you for reading this far! Even if that's all you've done – read the entire book, I guarantee your brain is already engaged in starting you on a new path to creating a healthier lifestyle. Honor yourself – start back at the beginning and commit to doing each Step.

If you took the time to actually practice each Step along the way – congratulations! I am even more proud of you! And thrilled that you found this information useful.

Keep going until all ten Steps (at any level) are part of your daily routine. You have the power to live a vibrant and productive life by making healthy choices a habit, one simple step at a time.

Be good to you.
Your body will thank you.

ABOUT THE AUTHOR

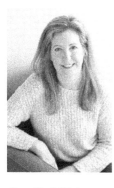

MAIR HILL has always been passionate about helping others through teaching, coaching and mentoring. Mair graduated *cum laude* from Colby College and at 25, started her own sales agency.

Now that her boys are grown, Mair is in the process of reinventing herself; starting a new chapter with her first love – health and wellness through personal transformation. She is a graduate of the Institute for Integrative Nutrition® and is a Certified Holistic Health Coach and Reiki Master

Always a multi-passionate entrepreneur, Mair is enjoying the process of inspiring others through a wide range of mediums: consulting, speaking, blogging, one-on-one coaching, social media and now writing her first book.

Mair grew up on both coasts and currently resides in the Chicago area with her husband, Rich. They have been beautifully married for almost forty years.

Mair Hill

www.MairHill.com
Facebook.com/mairhillinspires
Instagram: @mairhillinspires

CPSIA information can be obtained
at www.ICGtesting.com
Printed in the USA
BVHW031035271019
561909BV00001BA/1/P